Assistive Technology

in Special Education and Rehabilitation

Susan Sze, Ph.D.
Peter Cowden, Ph.D.
Niagara University

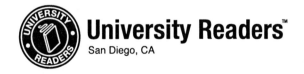

Copyright © 2009 by Susan Sze and Peter Cowden.
No part of this publication may be reproduced, stored in a retrieval system, or transmitted, in any form or by any means, without permission in writing from the publisher. University Readers is NOT affiliated or endorsed by any university or institution.

First published in the United States of America in 2009 by University Readers

13 12 11 10 09   1 2 3 4 5

Printed in the United States of America

ISBN: 978-1-934269-66-4

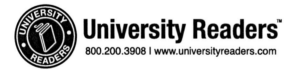

"Ever child needs to belong. …
Every child needs to be included …
It is our task to make this happen."

—Susan Sze

Contents

Introduction	1
PART I: A CRASH COURSE IN ASSISTIVE TECHNOLOGY	5
Section One	
Technology for Persons with Disabilities	7
Section Two	
Consideration of Special Factors in Development of IEP	9
Section Three	
Assistive Technology Device and Service	13
Section Four	
Low Tech, Med Tech, High Tech	15
PART II: LANGUAGE	17
Section Five	
Reading	19
Section Six	
Writing	25
Section Seven	
Composing Writing Material	29
Section Eight	
Communication	33
Section Nine	
Computer Access	37

PART III: MATH   **41**
   Section Ten
     Math   43

PART IV: LEARNING AND STUDYING   **51**
   Section Eleven
     Learning and Studying   53

PART V: SENSORY   **59**
   Section Twelve
     Vision   61
   Section Thirteen
     Hearing   67

PART VI: MOTOR   **71**
   Section Fourteen
     Control the Environment   73
   Section Fifteen
     Positioning and Seating   77
   Section Sixteen
     Mobility   79
   Section Seventeen
     Activities of Daily Living (ADLs)   83
   Section Eighteen
     Recreation   91

PART VII: TOP TEN   **95**
   Section Nineteen
     Approximately $1 Toolbox   97
   Section Twenty
     Resources   101

Introduction

Preface

Educators, parents, and other professionals who work with exceptional children search for a single comprehensive resource for assistive technology. This handbook goes a long way in fulfilling this need. This manual is a result of weeks of research and preparation by the graduate students under the direction of Dr. Susan Sze at Niagara University. It is the intent of the manual to provide a highly useful resource to teachers and others who work with students with disabilities. This handbook provides relevant information for caregivers as well as people with a wide array of disabilities.

"Raising a child with a disability presents families and professionals with many challenges. Today, one of the major challenges facing people who care for and about children and youth with disabilities is technology—what to get, where to get it, how to use it, how to pay for it, how to evaluate its effectiveness, and where to put it" (NICHCY, 1996).

Why Do You Need this Manual?

Differentiation, universal design, and inclusion—these educational methodologies depicting today's classroom are here to stay. What does the average general education teacher do to make sure that their students receive the best education? Where should a teacher turn to have a quick reference check for the usage of assistive technology? A manual such as this can provide not only exciting new ideas and equipment in the world of assistive technology, but the confidence in knowing that assistive technology is constantly being explored to best serve our students.

What is here today is gone tomorrow in the world of technology. It is important to be vigilant in an effort to maintain an on-going commitment to update your assistive technology and practices. Whereas the authors attempt to guide the reader into basic knowledge and information on assistive technology, it is the responsibility of the reader to continue to make inquiries for future reference.

The Assistive Technology Manual provides individuals with a broad presentation consisting of definitions, categories, purposes, and functional applications of assistive technology (AT) in relation to students' specialized educational programs. This AT Manual presents knowledge associated with specialty areas of assistive technology (e.g., access, alternative/augmentative communication, computer-based instruction, mobility, positioning, assistive listening and signaling devices, recreation/leisure/play, vision technology, environmental control, and activities of daily living). Furthermore, this collaborative resource assists individuals in applying discipline specific knowledge to the appropriate AT in a variety of educational settings. Therefore, this particular manual recognizes the need for ongoing individual professional development and maintaining knowledge of emerging technologies.

How to Use this Book

Teachers in both regular education and special education are always facing new challenges while attempting to meet the needs of students with special needs. Some of these students may have disabilities that require the use of some type of assistive technology. The technology used may range from very complex to surprisingly basic and simple. This helpful handbook briefly and accurately describes the different tools and techniques available to educators today. The book may be used as a quick reference for busy teachers who want a concise explanation of assistive technology that they can utilize in their classroom. New teachers or teachers with little experience in dealing with students with disabilities will find this handbook a very useful resource.

As you read this handbook, keep in mind that it was written by teachers for teachers and that there are some ideas that may be adapted to your own personal preference. When you find a technique or piece of technology that works well for your students you may want to highlight it for future reference. This easy to read handbook can be kept on hand in the classroom and since it is intentionally written in a clear, simple style it can be used to accommodate students as they are experiencing a problem in class. Many of the practical tips included in the book can be followed with little confusion. Some of the sections in this book include lists of valuable web sites that may be accessed in order to find more detailed explanations of the assistive technology that you are interested in. We encourage you to visit these sites which have helped provide some of the material for this handbook. It would also be beneficial to maintain an on-going list of updated web sites.

How this Book Is Organized

This book is organized to give the user the easiest access to information on assistive technology. The book is designed to give the reader the most up to date information on assistive technology. The handbook covers all areas of assistive technology. The book is categorized by topics, followed by *Sections* describing the devices.

The handbook begins with a basic introduction into assistive technology by answering such questions as what is assistive technology, why do we need assistive technology, and what are the differences in assistive technology. This handbook is designed to answer the basic questions about assistive technology first and then look at the individual devices more in depth.

The next part of the handbook looks at the types of devices for assistive technology when dealing with language. The sections are categorized by reading, writing, communication, and computer access. All the Sections' are divided into categories describing the specific devices.

The next part of the handbook deals with math and assistive technology. The user can look at any type of device and learn how it can used to improve math skills for the student. Learning and studying follows math and gives individuals' ideas on how to use assistive technology to improve study habits.

Sensory is the next topic that the handbook discusses. The sub-categories discussing sensory needs are vision and hearing. The handbook user can find information on any number of devices to help students that have hearing and vision difficulties

Motor skills make up the next part of the handbook for assistive technology. There are five Sections in the book dealing with motor skills. The sub-topics are controlling the environment, position and seating, mobility, activities of daily living, and recreation.

The final part of the handbook discusses devices that can be found for under $1.00. This part of the book is great for finding inexpensive ways to help improve learning. Following the items under a dollar section is the resource section. The resource section is divided into three categories: books, journals, and internet sites.

This book is user friendly and gives brief descriptions of each topic for the reader, which saves time when trying to decide which device is best for you and your students.

Where Do We Go from Here?

> Don't be afraid to give your best to what seemingly are small jobs. Every time you conquer one it makes you that much stronger. If you do the little jobs well, the big ones will tend to take care of themselves.
>
> —Dale Carnegie

These words ring true for the new discoveries in assistive technology. What might seem easy and manageable for someone without a disability might seem monumental for a person with a disability. Assistive technology can help a person with a disability become a happier and more self-fulfilled person. We need to continue with our exploration of AT to better the lives of all persons needing help.

—Susan Sze PhD

Part I: A Crash Course in Assistive Technology

Section One

TECHNOLOGY FOR PERSONS WITH DISABILITIES

What Is Assistive Technology?

Assistive technology (AT) is a term used to describe any piece of equipment, from the simplest to the most complex, that is modified or customized, and can be used to increase or maintain current functional capabilities of individuals with disabilities. Examples of such technology could include special grips for holding utensils or various types of computer software such as voice recognition and screen reader capabilities. A student with a disability can use assistive technology to complete a task easier, faster, or in a better way while increasing independence.

Why Is It Important for All Educators to Be Aware of Assistive Technology?

Assistive technology can significantly improve the quality of life of a student with disabilities for better learning, independence, and life functions.

Who Will Benefit from Assistive Technology?

Assistive equipment enhances the ability of students and employees to be more efficient and successful while living with a disability. For individuals that are classified with LD, computer grammar checkers, an overhead projector used by a teacher, or the audiovisual information delivered through a CD-ROM would be typical examples. Devices to control the environment could be necessary for a child with severe or multiple physical disabilities who have limited ability to move about, such as seating and positioning devices for help with functioning and accessing the environment. Other types of equipment could include communication devices for speech and hearing impairments ...

Section Two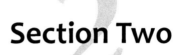

CONSIDERATION OF SPECIAL FACTORS IN DEVELOPMENT OF IEP

The Law and Assistive Technology

The Education for the Handicapped Act was reauthorized in 1997 as the Individuals with Disabilities Education Act, which now specifically addresses the inclusion of assistive technology in the IEP. The regulations specify that: (1) The need for assistive technology must be addressed on every IEP(2) Assistive technology can be special education or a related service that is necessary in order for the student to benefit from his or her education (3) Assistive technology can also be a form of supplemental aid or service utilized to facilitate a student's education in a regular education environment, or in the least restrictive environment possible and (4) If participants on the IEP team determine that a student requires assistive technology and if the device or services is needed for the student to make meaningful educational progress designating the device as either assistive technology or a related service then the services must be provided at no cost to the parents.

IEP Assessment

IDEA '97 requires that IEP teams "consider whether the child requires assistive technology devices and services." This means that all teams need to address whether assistive technology is required for the child to benefit from public education. It goes on to suggest that the team needs to determine what type of device or service is required. Districts must provide AT necessary to provide a free and appropriate public education. This technology is not required to be the best available.

AT Procedure

There are forms designed to provide IEP teams with a conceptual framework for assistive technology considerations that will be either too expansive or restrictive. In addition, the forms provide an option for documenting assistive technology considerations to satisfy the IEP requirements of IDEA. The forms are organized into the areas of:

- Reading
- Writing
- Access to educational programs
- Math
- Listening
- Orientation/mobility/ambulation
- Study skills
- Transition
- Speech/language
- Daily living/recreation/leisure

If a student has instructional, developmental or access needs in one or more of these areas, the IEP team can use the corresponding forms to assist in their consideration of a variety of assistive technology devices and services to address that area. To the greatest extent possible, teachers must ensure that assistive technology devices are embedded in IEPs. Assistive technology provides a means for including children with disabilities in a wide range of activities that might otherwise be unavailable or inaccessible to them.

The SETT framework provides a model IEP teams could use to select the most appropriate AT. SETT is an acronym that stands for student, environment, tasks, and tools. Once the team has sufficient data to acknowledge the student's individual strengths and weaknesses, the environment (s) the student works in, and the tasks needed to complete assignments along with the tools and skills; the team can better decide the most effective AT on an individual basis.

Links

http://www.pluk.org/AT1.html
www.ldonline.org/ld_indepth/technology/at-iep.html

Section Three

ASSISTIVE TECHNOLOGY DEVICE AND SERVICE

Define Purpose and Application

The most important underlying concept in providing assistive technology services and devices to students with special needs is to define the purpose and application it has to the individual student and how it can be incorporated into various educational programs. These services and devices can be integrated into home and school activities to assist everyday living such as computer-based instruction, assistive listening and signaling devices, vision technology and environmental control.

Teachers need to realize that AT can be applied to a variety of disciplines to service students with special needs. Teachers may want to start by deciding the setting specific needs of their classroom, and the requisite abilities needed to be successful in order to determine specific AT that may be needed for an individual student. Parents should also be included as team members in the process of determining the AT to be used, and other school staff members should be utilized to better assist individual students. Special education instructors should work in a team setting with other school staff members that are directly involved in the daily education of a student and make certain that all the needs of the student are met. Teachers also need to be aware of where and when to refer to various resources when they do not hold the necessary knowledge.

IEP Consideration and AT

Assistive technology should be integrated into IEPs based upon individual student strengths, tasks and expectations that work best with the ability of the student. A formal IEP should include the various AT devices, services and strategies that the student requires. Team members should discuss available AT resources in the classroom, school building, school district, region, community, state and national level, funding, product resources, print and electronic resources, human resources (specialty teachers and training) and problem solving if something wrong should occur (repair). Team members working with students with special needs should assess each individual student requiring AT in customary environments and formal reports and recommendations should be made on continual basis. Teams should also consider possible AT needed to allow independence in every day living skills outside of the school setting.

Validity

After the IEP plan that includes AT is implemented, team members should validate, evaluate, measure and report progress and effectiveness of the plan, modifying if necessary. This process should take place on a continual basis; the team will need to consider what data should be collected to determine the student's progress. All members of the team should be in constant contact throughout the entire school year.

Section Four

LOW TECH, MED TECH, HIGH TECH

Low Technology

Low-tech items are less sophisticated and generally low cost. They can include devices such as adapted spoon handles, non-tipping drinking cups, Velcro fasteners, pencil grips, magnifiers, special paper or a walking cane or crutches. For a visually impaired child, raised lines on a piece of paper could be helpful, while for students who need OT services, weighted pencils or a rubber tip to help turn pages in a book could be beneficial. Students can often be taught an assistive behavior to manage a challenging task and to eventually gain full independence. For example, instead of buying an expensive medium technology mixer, a student can be taught to wedge the bowl between the counter and their hip and be successful.

Medium Technology

Medium-tech devices are relatively complicated mechanical devices, such as wheelchairs, walkers, calculators, talking devices, a print enhancement device, tape recorder or microphone.

High Technology

High-tech devices incorporate sophisticated electronics or computers. Due to the many varying degrees of disabilities there are a variety of products available to users. One example is a screen reader to assist a student with low vision by providing speech output and magnification for them. A Text to Speech program will read each word out loud as the student types. Another example includes switches available to students with little strength and mobility. Also for students with low strength and mobility is an eye tracking system which moves the cursor according to the user's eye movement. There are other high technology devices available according to your student's personal need.

Varied Use of Technology

A varied use of technology combing all three identified above may be helpful for; a student with a disability in building social interaction, attention, expressive communication and independent daily skills. Any technology that is chosen should be utilized daily and routinely, especially for students diagnosed with Learning Disabilities, autism, or mental retardation.

Part II: Language

Section Five

READING

Predictable Books

Predictable books make use of rhyme, repetition of words, phrases, sentences and refrains, and such patterns as cumulative structure, repeated scenes, familiar cultural sequences, interlocking structure and turnaround plots. These stories invite children to make predictions or guesses about words, phrases, sentences, events and characters that could come next in the story. Types of predictable books could include a circular story in which the ending of the reading leads back to the beginning, or a cumulative story in which all past events are repeated every time another event begins.

The use of predictable books is critical to the scaffolding process of reading. Assistive technology can be employed with predictable genre of literature. *Tape recordings* can be purchased or created by the teacher to be used in *listening centers*. Students can listen and follow along with the words in the book. After the predictable story has been introduced and students are familiar with the pattern the rhythm the teacher could also *play the tape for entire class read/ listen along*. The *overhead projector* can be a helpful tool when setting the introduction and purpose of the predicable book. The use of an introductory poem or skill building materials can be shared with the whole class. An excellent source for information on predictable books is www.earlyliterature.ecsd.net.

Changes in Text Size, Spacing, Color, and Background

Some students may have trouble: following the lines of text (where words jump or move on the page), decoding complex words, or scanning text for important information. There are low and mid tech tools that can help with compensating for these difficulties.

1. Text size—Changing the size of the text can help individuals with vision problems. Larger font enables the learner to see the material. Students with decoding problems can benefit from larger text size as well.
2. Spacing—Providing text that is double spaced helps the learner to follow the lines of text without jumping to the line above or below.
3. Color—Colored transparent sheets placed over a page of black and white text help the person with visual processing problems. Often these individuals complain that the text jumps, moves, or swirls on the page. The color overlay choice is individualized to the person seeing the text. Frequently it is by trial and error that the person discovers which color helps them see the words easily. These rulers can also be used to track reading.
4. Highlighting—The students who have problems with scanning the text for important information can benefit from highlighting. Using a variety of colors helps the person code the text for corresponding information. This helps students with study skills (5) Background—Changing the color of the background for some students aids them in their reading. The stark contrast between the black text and white page may not be as visible as black text on a colored background. Changing the background of a computer screen can also help these students.

Books Adapted for Page Turning

Page turning can be facilitated for an individual with low dexterity. This kind of impairment results from having limited or low finger, hand, or arm dexterity. The first method involves a low tech accommodation where the pages of books have Velcro for easier page turning. Another adaptation utilizes the use of switch activated devices for page turning. Many low dexterity individuals can activate machines using an electric switch. For example, one company, Resna, offers such people a low cost device that allows users to turn a page of printed material by simply touching a switch with their head, hands, or other body parts. Thus, individuals with low dexterity are granted more independence and can enjoy increased interaction with books and other printed media. Or, the company GEWA offers a more advanced and expensive program that will even go as far as turning pages backwards for its reader.

Use of Pictures/Symbols with Text

One of the areas of assistive technology that has really expanded has been the use of software that is capable of creating visual supports for children that require it. It is important to provide children with autism and other developmental disorders with visually supported materials to increase their understanding of their environment and behavior expectations.

Boardmaker and PictureIt are two software programs used for these purposes. Boardmaker is a database with 3000 graphic picture communication symbols (PCS). Picture It develops stories or directions that include text and accompanying pictures to give visual opportunities to expand individual success to emergent readers, students with pervasive developmental disorders, autism, English as a second language, learning disabilities, developmental disorders, hearing impairments, and children with cognitive impairments,. Following the development of symbol-processing software there has been an explosion of symbol-enhanced teaching materials in special schools. These materials have provided many students with opportunities to enhance their learning by making information around the school accessible. Teaching resources such as flash cards, worksheets, timetables, age appropriate reading books and communication books can be produced relatively quickly and easily through the use of the adaptive software.

Talking Electronic Device to Speak Challenging Words

There are several computer software programs which read text aloud. Some software applications read the text within their own software; other applications can be paired with separate software in order to have the text read aloud. For example, READPLEASE is a freeware program that reads aloud text copied into its own window. NATURAL READER is yet another example of a free download made available through Microsoft. Certainly there are many options for assistive technology that do not affect the pocketbook.

Single Word Scanners

Small devices are available for people with learning disabilities and dyslexia. These pens scan the material, speak aloud the word, give the definition, and display the word on their small screen. These devices include a complete dictionary to help not only those with reading difficulties, but also English language learners. One such device is called the *Reading Pen Oxford*; another is the *Wizcom Scanner Pen*.

Scanner with Optical Character Recognition and Talking Word Processor

There has been an explosion of symbol-enhanced teaching materials in special schools. Optical Character Recognition (OCR) allows educators the opportunity to scan text in a number of languages to assist students with reading difficulties. Then you can hear this text read out loud to you. It is possible to use Optical Character Recognition (OCR) to scan documents and books to get information into a computer without having to type it in or spell it. A Text-to-Speech package can then be used to read it out. For individuals with dyslexia or vision problems who find reading very difficult or tiring, this may be easier than reading with their own eyes, but it is a laborious process. The more expensive packages make it much quicker and easier by doing the scan OCR read at once. If you are doing a significant amount of scanning this is a much better solution. Scanners generally include a light version of an OCR package in the box to get you started. This light version may be enough for very casual use, but the full product will give optimal results.

OpenBook software is one example. This program allows you to convert printed documents or graphic based text into an electronic text format using accurate optical character recognition and quality speech. Its low vision tools allow you to customize how the document appears on your screen, while other features provide portability. It also provides the flexibility to use either of the two text to speech software synthesizers: RealSpeak and Via Voice. RealSpeak features a natural, human-sounding voice that can help enhance your reading experience. This program also supports most hardware speech synthesizers.

OmniPage Pro is another type of scanning software that uses optical character recognition (OCR) to scan printed pages into a readable and editable format. You can scan letters, newspapers, books, magazines, and other printed material directly into applications such as Microsoft Word. The RealSpeak Text-to-Speech feature included in OmniPage Pro enables you to hear recognized texts read aloud.

Electronic Books

Electronic books are available for use on the computer. They can be downloaded from the Internet, usually for a fee, and read on a computer. E-books can also be downloaded into small PDA's that are easy to carry. Font, color, and text size can be adjusted on many of these books to assist in the reading of the text.

Section Six

WRITING

Variety of Pencils and Pens

Sometimes the best AT options may be low- tech or no tech—options without any "bells and whistles". Writing skills can often be enhanced by using simple methods or devices. Simple adaptations, like smooth writing pens can make the difference between needing physical assistance and working independently. Pens or pencils with thicker barrels may be easier to hold on to and have a broad enough point to make a wide line that can hide unsteady writing. Colored pens are available to provide visual emphasis for those who may need it as well as a pen with a flashlight built into the top barrel. Teachers should keep in mind that erasable pens make corrections easy and gel pens may glide easier. In order to accommodate the varying needs of students, it is a wise technique to provide a variety of writing tools in order to best assist each individual.

Pencil/Pen with Adaptive Grip

Pencil grips come in a variety of shapes, sizes, and colors. They are slipped onto pens and pencils to provide a stable holding surface for individuals who are right or left handed. Some pens have grips built in. Pencil grips can help some kids with fine motor skill problems or writing difficulties take control. Some students can more easily grasp and hold pens, pencils or markers if they're built up and made larger. There are several non-slip grips on the market that can help. Students can even slide a foam roller over a pencil grip to make it bigger still. For a customized fit, some teachers have even wrapped a small amount of modeling clay around the writing tool. When the student places his or her hand around it he or she will create a customized hand mold with the writing utensil. The following website offers ideas for a huge variety of grip solutions: www.pencilgrip.com.

Slant Boards

A slant board provides a smooth, angled, "drafting table" work surface that helps position the wrist for writing. It can be made of plastic, wood, or even cardboard. Some provide padded arm support. Other teachers simply use an empty three-ring binder turned with the rings facing away from the student. This helps visually and mechanically with writing and is easy to carry.

Templates

Templates are used as a way to focus students on a particular concept, create a report, or jumpstart their thinking in some way. A template provides a framework for directed learning, and the teacher can design the template to enhance and extend classroom learning across the curriculum. Templates can also be used for open-ended, creative projects in all subject areas. The teacher can provide a story starter, or have the student begin with a set of minimum requirements.

Prewritten Words/Phrases

Some students may not have the motor skills necessary for using traditional pencil and paper. One way to provide them with the opportunity to produce written work is to use prewritten words or phrases that can be placed in sentences and paragraphs.

A low-tech way to do this is with adhesive backed magnetic labels or strips. Words can be pre printed on paper or card stock and stuck to the magnetic material. The student can then arrange them on a metal surface such as a cookie sheet. There are also software programs that facilitate writing words and phrases before the student is ready to spell individual words or to keyboard.

Portable Word Processor

Portable word processors can be an exceptionally effective tool to support students who are struggling with writing. Whether the student uses a portable word processor or a fully functioning computer, these tools offer the opportunity to change letters, words, sentences and paragraphs easily and quickly while allowing a clean, attractive and readable product. Some of these products also interface with a computer for printing and/or storage of the students work.

Computer with Word Processing

Computers with word processors are often used for students with disabilities. It is an important application of assistive technology for students of this population. As most of these students are identified as needing assistance in language arts, particularly in their writing skills, the use of computers and word processing software, can help students formulate ideas on paper without the impediment imposed by writing with paper and pencil. Computers also have grammar and spell checkers, dictionaries, and thesauruses which are tools to help assist children in the mechanics of writing. Lastly, computers with word processing are beneficial to the editing process because they eliminate problems such as torn papers, poor handwriting, lost papers, and the final copies are always neat and legible.

Voice Recognition Software

Voice recognition software is used to assist students who have learning disabilities that interfere with their ability to spell, write or even manipulate a standard keyboard. The visual-motor demands of using a keyboard can be a major stumbling block that compounds the writing process. If students' oral motor abilities far exceed their ability to generate text with pencil and paper or the standard word processing, voice recognition may enable them to become successful writers.

Talking Calculators

A talking calculator has a built in speech synthesizer that reads aloud each number, symbol, operation key the user presses; it also vocalizes the answer. This auditory feedback may help someone who also struggles in math. Talking calculators are used to benefit students with vision impairments. Visually impaired students may not be able to see the numbers on the calculator, but the calculator can talk back to them and tell them what buttons they are pushing and the answer they got.

http://www.schools.pinellas.k12.fl.us/tchandbk/Assttech1.htm
http://schwablearning.org/articles.aspx?r=1076

Section Seven

COMPOSING WRITING MATERIAL

Word Cards/Book/Wall

Word cards/book/wall is an excellent way to help students with special needs to learn vocabulary without having the added pressure of straining to look at a word wall from across the room. Students who are visually impaired should be placed next to a word wall or be given a word book or word cards that define the vocabulary words that are to be studied for that day/week. In this way, students with special needs are concentrating on learning the words as opposed to having to strain to look at the word or hear the teacher say the word. Enlarged print of vocabulary words and definitions also aids in students with vision impairments.

Pocket Dictionary/Thesaurus

A pocket dictionary/thesaurus is an effective way to help students look up definitions without having to flip through a large dictionary to find one word. This device is most useful for students with difficulty with fine and gross motor skills, attention deficit disorders, learning disabilities, and traumatic brain injuries. With a pocket dictionary, students are able to easily look through the dictionary for a given word. When students are using a pocket dictionary it may be helpful for students to have labels at the beginning of each letter to easily identify where each section in the dictionary begins.

Writing Templates

Writing templates can be most useful for students who take longer time to complete assignments and who forget to complete a proper heading on each paper. It is useful to help students with disabilities with organization and to get their thoughts in order on paper. With a template, students are able to concentrate on the assignment itself as opposed to having the proper format; which serve as distractions to students with disabilities. With a writing template, students become familiar and learn the format of writing assignments. They can just simply concentrate on the given assignment and getting words on paper. For the majority of students with disabilities requiring AT services and devices, the main problem is either physical writing or the inability to clearly get words down on paper.

Electronic/Talking Spell Checker/Dictionary

An electronic/talking spell checker/dictionary is a great way to aid students with fine and gross motor skills and those with reading and or vision problems. An electronic method to check words enables students to quickly check their work without the time and frustration of having to locate words in a large dictionary that is difficult to handle. This method enables students to check their work, and is easily used by students and requires little training.

Word Processing with Spell Checker

As with the electronic/talking spell checker, a word processor with a spell checker enables students with reading and/or fine and gross motor skills to quickly and easily check their work while doing the assignment. Without the word processor with spell checker, students with disabilities will have to locate a hard copy of a dictionary to refer to for all misspelled words. They first need to have their paper proofread by a teacher. With a spell checker on the word processor, students with disabilities will be able to see their mistakes on the computer and the spell checker will make the corrections. This saves much time and energy since the device is convenient. Students can also see how misspelled words are correctly spelled for future reference.

Talking Word Processing

These systems are designed to help individuals that have trouble reading and writing. Talking word processing is a text to speech system where students can compose written material. Talking word processing highlights and reads the words, sentences and paragraphs. This device provides both audio and visual support to the student while helping the student learn and recognize new vocabulary. It allows the users to hear words and become familiar with how those words are said. Talking word processing allows the user to see the words or sentences being spoken, which helps expand spelling ability.

Abbreviation/Expansion

Abbreviation and expansion systems allow the typist to use two, three or more characters for typing phrases and sentences (Gilman, 2002). The systems are designed to cut down on the amount of letters a person needs to type to complete a sentence or phrase. A person must first assign abbreviations to a particular sentence or phrase in order for the software to recognize the abbreviation. The user then types in the abbreviation and the sentence or phrase appears. Abbreviation/Expansion could be useful for students with various learning disabilities.

Word Processing with Writing Support

Word processing systems with writing support are designed to help students produce written work. Word prediction is a software system that assists individuals who struggle with spelling and grammar. Word prediction tries to guess or "predict" the word you are about to type. The system provides a drop down screen and the user picks a word from the screen that best fits the word that person was looking for. The system is a great tool for expanding vocabulary and for helping to improve spelling.

Multimedia Software

Multimedia software is designed to help students with disabilities find alternative ways to access and represent knowledge and information. Effective multimedia software can vary depending on the need of the student and can be used in a variety of ways to help enhance the students' ability to learn. Multimedia tools can range from simple graphics to the integration of text, graphics, video, music, and sound effects. (NCIP Library) Often, multimedia software can help the student compose writing while making it interesting to the student by using a combination of graphics, video, and sound effects that are found on the software.

Voice Recognition Software

Voice recognition enables users to control their computers through speech. Students who have great difficulty writing and learning to use a keyboard can use voice recognition software. Users speak into a microphone and can tell the computer to execute commands. Students can also write using voice recognition in conjunction with a standard word processing program. The words appear on the screen as the users say them in a word processing format. The accuracy rate of voice recognition software can be as high as 98%. The users must take the time to properly train and use the voice recognition software, as the system will never be 100% accurate. This device could be beneficial for students with poor or low motor skills.

Section Eight

COMMUNICATION

Communication Board with Pictures/Words/Objects

A communication board is a simple augmentative communication device. A communication board is made of cardboard or felt and created with pictures, words, or letters. A communication board provides an avenue for communication for an individual with language difficulties.

Eye Gaze Frame

The eye gaze frame is an eye controlled word processor. This technique is used to track the gaze of a person by probing into subjects' perceptual or cognitive processes in order to measure eye movements. For example, tracking can be done during driving in traffic or reading text. Some eye tracking techniques use contact lenses which can be so obtrusive that they cannot be used for extensive periods. Some techniques have been made totally unobtrusive and allow for (small) head movements, making them usable for enhancing the user-interfaces for individuals with disabilities especially quadriplegics.

Simple Voice Output Device

Simple voice output device is a communication aid that provides a large target area for an individual to press for a single recorded message. Some allow even those with the most limited communication abilities to carry on an essential conversation, or give a series of instructions, conduct an interview, or express a single message in a variety of ways.

Voice Output Device with Icon Sequencing

There are a variety of voice output devices with icon sequencing. A few voice output devices with icon sequencing are (1) Alphatlker II, (2) Liberator II, and (3) Chatbox.

1. The Alphatalker II uses an introductory vocabulary program. It is easy to use and offers: icon prediction, auditory scanning/feedback cues so that persons with visual impairments can know what location is being activated, and environmental control commands. The digitized speech allows the user to record anyone's voice.
2. The Liberator II gives words we use everyday and words we need for specific situations. It offers electronic notebooks for writing papers, letters, and list.
3. The ChatBox voice is designed any individual who experiences cognitive and language limitations, brain disorders, cerebral palsy or conditions that result in temporary loss of speech. The ChatBox can be programmed for the appropriate vocabulary, voice and native tongue of the user. It can be utilized effectively by individuals of any age as a primary aid to daily communication or as a "first" communication aid from which one transitions to a more flexible system. ChatBox is an affordable, entry-level device which introduces a non-speaking individual to electronic voice aids.

These devices provide word prediction, math scratch pad and calculator, clock, calendar, and alarm notification, auditory scanning and feedback. By organizing vocabulary around activities and situations, the beginning aided communicator is provided with sufficient vocabulary for use at home, school, work or play.

Voice Output Device with Dynamic Display

Voice output devices with dynamic display are: (1) DynaMytes and (2) DynaVox.

The DynaMyte is a powerful, easy-to-carry communication device. It offers fast processing speed, communication and page creation. It uses dynamic "touch-screen" display to allow communicators to move smoothly through the same natural message-formation process that produces normal speech.

The DynaVox device has the same features as the DynaMyte except that it provides a larger screen for more vocabulary and weighs 7 pounds. One can access a DynaVox by touching it, using a mouse-compatible input device, switch joystick, or scanning. Visual and auditory scanning allows individuals, who need to activate a switch using one controllable movement, access to the full range of the DynaVox.

Voice Output Devices with Speech Synthesis

Some types of voice output devices that rely on spelling are: (1) LightWRITER and (2) Link.

1. LightWRITERs are text to speech devices and require some degree of literacy for users who suffer from acquired speech loss following laryngectomy, tracheostomy, head injury, stroke, or with progressive neurological diseases such as ALS, Parkinson's Disease, or Multiple Sclerosis. This device is very portable and unique in having dual displays, one facing the user so they can see what they are typing, and a second outfacing display to allow communication in a natural face-to-face position.
2. The Link is a keyboard and a communication device. Link are text to speech devices and require some degree of literacy and note-taking ability. It is easy to use, lightweight, and transportable. The Link features abbreviation expansion and "instant messages" to make communicating easy and fast. The device saves files that can be downloaded to any Macintosh or PC computer.

Section Nine

COMPUTER ACCESS

Keyboard with Accessibility Options

Modern versions of Windows provide a number of accessibility features that are designed to make the system easier to use for those with special needs. Several of these are related to the operation of the keyboard. All of these function at the operating system level and so work transparently to virtually all software. Some options are: Sticky Keys, when enabled, this function causes modifier keys to "stick" until they are either manually released, or until a keystroke combination is complete. Filter Keys suppress or ignore bursts of keystrokes that are sent too quickly--either fast streams of the same key or clumps of different keys sent all at once. Such bursts might, for example, be made by someone who does not have perfect control of his or her fingers due to a tremor. A number of settings let you control how long a key must be held down for it to register, set audible confirmations and other options. Toggle Keys provides an audible indication when any of the permanent (locking) modifier keys is pressed.

Word Prediction

Word prediction software programs have been available for IBM and Macintosh personal computer for several years. The concept of word prediction began as a simple assistive tool to reduce the number of keystrokes necessary for individuals with mobility impairment, making it easier to communicate and less fatiguing for the user.

Keyguard

A keyguard is a plexiglass cover for a keyboard with holes for the individual keys. A keyguard allows for a more precise selection of keys for an individual with fine motor difficulties.

Arm Support

The arm support enables the user to use the mouse without lifting an arm off the rest. For computing, it brings the mouse up to same level as the keyboard. It provides comfortable arm, shoulder and neck support with unrestricted motion. The arm support can aid people with gross motor difficulties or individuals with arm, shoulder or neck injuries.

Track Ball/Joystick

The track ball and/or joystick is a replacement for the mouse pointing device that uses a rolling ball to perform mouse tasks. This tool assists individuals who have difficulty with movement of their hands, wrists or arms.

Alternate Keyboard

An alternative keyboard may include enlarged, reduced, varied key placement, one-handed, Braille, chordic, or any other device for entering text on a computer. This device might be used by individuals with poor motor skills or coordination or individuals who are missing a hand or limb.

Computer Access

Pointing Options/Head Mice

A head mouse is a type of pointing option that replaces the standard desktop computer mouse. A head mouse is a device that can translate the movements of a user's head into directly proportional movements of the computer mouse pointer. A head mouse sensor replaces the standard desktop computer mouse for people who cannot use their hands. This device will track the user's head with the user located in any comfortable viewing position relative to the computer display. This device is very precise and allows a user to perform tasks such as drawing or Computer Aided Design.

Switch with Morse Code

Morse Code is a direct method for computer input using one to three switches and coded input to replace the keyboard and mouse. Switches with Morse Code may be used by an individual with severe motor difficulties by any controllable muscle in their body (head, hand, toe, eye, breath, etc.) to operate any type of computer, communication or environmental control device.

Switch with Scanning

Scanning is another method for accessing a computer or communication device using one or more switches. Scanning involves presenting a group of choices, cycling among them and making choices by activating a switch. Once again, this system may be used by an individual with severe motor difficulties by any controllable muscle in their body.

Voice Recognition Software

Voice recognition software uses a microphone that allows input and control with voice commands. This software would be helpful to an individual with motor difficulties.

Part III: Math

Section Ten

MATH

Introduction

Math symbols are a way to express numerical language concepts. This makes language skills very important to learning math. In addition, many students with a learning disability in reading have a difficult time solving word problems which can lead to low self esteem. This can inhibit the student's ability to apply math concepts, lead to math phobias and avoidance behaviors. Assistive technology can help students compensate for many of the areas they are struggling with.

Abacus/Math Line

Mathline allows the learner to see the relation between the concrete methods of mathematics and the abstract symbols used to represent numbers. This learning tool allows the student to use manipulatives in an organized manner. By using this tool, the student has less of a chance of losing the traditional manipulatives or losing track of the counting during the mathematical process. Mathline is similar to the ideas used in an abacus. This math concept also allows the student to remain organized and visualize the math processes in a self contained tool.

Enlarged Math Worksheets

Students with LD often get frustrated with the excessive amount of information on any given worksheet or test. Symbol discrimination is often challenging in many current math programs. Helpful strategies include minimizing the amount of problems per page, enlarge the page, as well as keeping the worksheets one sided. The enlarged sheet and reducing the problems presents the information in smaller more manageable portions.

One sided papers reduce distraction and allows students to focus on the task at hand.

Alternatives for Answering, Explaining or Giving Examples

As an alternative for answering, explaining, or giving examples, a disabled student can use connecting cubes or straws (manipulatives) to represent the value of the data recorded on a hard copy, with the assistance of a partner. Visual representation for answers can help students who find it difficult to communicate orally.

Math "Smart Chart"

The Smart Chart provides an effective means of monitoring the skill levels of individual students. Teachers can use the data to pinpoint specific areas of the curriculum that need special attention. The chart can be printed to show parents their student's accomplishments or to reward students for their successes.

Money Calculator/Coin-u-lator

A coin-u-lator is a hand held calculator with realistic keys shaped and sized exactly like coins along with a smaller dollar bill. This technology piece allows students to add and subtract amounts of money as well as practice money skills. It can also include coordinating games to expand relevant learning. The coin-u-lator can be easily transported with the child to be utilized in promoting real life skills when shopping.

Tactile/Voice Output Measuring Devices

These talking measuring devices include such objects as rulers, clocks, and watches. There are even tire pressure gages that use a talking mechanism to tell the air pressure inside of a tire. Such devices help the individual who has trouble reading or seeing not only in the academic setting, but also with life skills.

Talking Watches/Clocks

Talking watches allow visually impaired individuals to tell time and set alarms for appointments and medication alerts. The wearer can also get voice feedback from the watch that allows the person to set the functions of the watch. There are also talking alarm clocks, vibrating clocks to help sleepers wake up and wall clocks with large numbers are also available for the visually impaired.

Calculator with or without Print Out

Calculators with or without print are low tech valuable tools. Students using calculators may have better attitudes towards mathematics and much better self-concepts in mathematics. The use of calculators does not impede on student ability to perform paper-and-pencil computational skills. Other content areas where improvement has been shown when these calculators have been used in instruction include function concepts and spatial visualization. Other studies have found that students are better problem solvers when using graphing calculators. In addition, students are more flexible in their thinking with regard to solution strategies, have greater perseverance and focus more on trying to understand the problem conceptually rather than simply focusing on computations.

Calculator with Large Keys and/or Display

Several different companies offer calculators with large keys and/or display. These calculators range from the basic four function to scientific calculators. Such devices allow the students with vision and dexterity difficulties the ability to manipulate and see the devices more easily.

Talking Calculator

Talking calculators are available for use in the classroom, workplace, and home. These calculators come in styles that allow the user to plug in an earphone so the people surrounding the user will not be disturbed. The calculator can be used for those people who need to focus their attention on the task at hand, as well as those with visual impairments. Features may include speaking the number as a unit instead of the individual digits, date and time announcements, and advanced calculations.

Calculator with Special Features

Calculators are such a common aspect of the math world that there are numerous calculators with special features on the market. Students with learning disabilities are at a great advantage in the current education setting. Some special features include:

>**Screen Emulator:** This is software which emulates graphing calculators on your home computer. The advantage of screen emulators is better visibility on a computer monitor over the conventional graphing calculator's smaller display for visually impaired or to minimize distraction and maximize concentration for the LD student.
>**Enlarging and Projecting Displays:** Devices enlarge and project images from a calculator so they can be viewed by a group or class, works with standard overhead projector and TV screen.
>**LED Display:** LED Calculators are often brighter, and easier to read than standard LCD calculators.
>**X-Large Display:** Numbers on the display are 1/2" high or larger.

Contrasting Keypad: The numbers on the keypads are a contrasting color than the keypad's color, making the numbers stand out better.

On-screen Scanning Calculator

One on-screen scanning calculator is *BigCalc*, from Don Johnson, Inc. Another is Calcu-scan. Products such as these allow the student to learn to use the computer and practice mathematical computations. Furthermore, this type of calculator allows the teacher to program in specific math problems, including word problems, for the student to work with.

Alternative Keyboard

Alternative keyboards help to reduce demands upon the hands and arms, improve posture, and prevent repetitive strain injuries. Some special features include:

(1) Vertical split keyboards take the traditional keyboard and place it upright. This helps to reduce carpal tunnel problems and other repetitive strain injuries.
(2) Chording keyboards are smaller and have fewer keys, typically one for each finger and possibly the thumbs. Each character requires multiple keys to be pushed. This allows for a smaller keyboard, but requires hours of training.
(3) Split keyboards allow the typist to adjust the keyboard to more comfortable positions to allow for ease of motion.
(4) Safe type keyboards allow the typist to use the device if there is limited reach capabilities.

Math Software

Math software is a very lucrative business. There are literally hundreds of software programs available on the market. It is a market where the educated consumer is his or her own best friend. When shopping for math software a teacher needs to understand the math curriculum for his or her district as well as the New York State Math Standards when purchasing an appropriate program to maximize the investment. Below is an example of a review company that offers assistance in informing the consumer.

Super Kids' reviewers compared five Math Software programs, evaluating their content and design, as well as their kid appeal and ease of use. Which is best for your child?

http://www.superkids.com/aweb/pages/reviews/math/4/sw_sum1.shtml

- Carmen Sandiego Math Detective [for ages 8 to 14] from Broderbund, provides fun math exercises wrapped in a mystery-solving story. Best for young child who already knows basic math facts.
- Math Quest with Aladdin [for ages 7 to 10] from Disney, is an Indiana Jones-like adventure, filled with math-based problem-solving activities. Best for young child who already knows basic math facts.
- Math for the Real World [for ages 10 and up] from Davidson, has the user traveling the countryside with a hot new rock band, making money to produce a video. Real-world, word problems.
- Number Maze Challenge [for ages 5 to 12] from Great Wave Software, offers 350 levels of math problems, by topic and grade level. Not much sizzle, but captivating to students interested in math and/or maze solving.
- School House Rock! 1s–4th Grade Math Essentials [for ages 6 to 10] from Creative Wonders, offers young students the opportunity to develop and practice multiple levels of math skills in cleverly designed challenges. Better-suited for the lower grade levels as it becomes complex and difficult to follow at higher levels.
- Timez Attack [for ages 7–10] from Big Brainz, Inc., a video game filled with multiplication and education. The value of numbers is illustrated as children solve multiplication problems that have been presented before, with special focus on problems that have proven difficult before. This program may be difficult for those who have difficulty with fine motor skills, and students may need some initial knowledge of multiplication.
- Transition Math [for ages 4–6] from School Zone Publishing, a worksheet type program that allows children to spend time individually solving problems. Children complete worksheets on basic math, with emphasis on important math terms, and are immediately given feedback on how they are

doing. This is not a program to be used if looking for critical thinking or open ended questions.

Software for Manipulation of Objects

IntelliTools is a software program that allows the student to use math manipulatives on the computer. Programs such as this allow the student with limited dexterity or mobility, or those who need other supportive devices, to use the computer instead of hand held manipulatives to learn concrete mathematical concepts. The program meets the accessibility requirements of section 508 of the Rehabilitation Act. This program can only be purchased in combination with IntellIiTools Classroom Suite.

Voice Recognition Software

Programs such as *Apple Speech Recognition* allow users to do addition, subtraction, division, and multiplication by voice. This particular program is designed for students in grades 1-5 and is designed to recognize speech immediately, without training the program. Other programs, such as *Virtual Pencil*, are designed to be used by those who are blind. This program helps the student to do the mathematical tasks that would normally be hand written. The program is designed to produce results in Braille or linked with a talking program. MathTalk is another voice activated program that can be used for students in grades 6 and up, including doctoral programs. Within Math Talk, there is a MathBrailleTalk program which is linked to a Duxbury Braille Translator so those who are visually impaired will be able to use their voice to create the Braille symbols.

Part IV: Learning and Studying

Section Eleven

LEARNING AND STUDYING

Print or Picture Schedule

Students with certain disabilities often have trouble with remembering and following instructions. They may have difficulty with organization, which is critical for effective learning and studying. To assist students with these difficulties, it is helpful to provide the student with a print or picture schedule. There is computer software available that may be used to create a visual schedule specifically designed for young people who may have difficulty verbalizing. The "boardmaker" places pictures in the place of words to create a daily schedule that is easy to interpret. Another piece of software links pictures with the words that are typed into the computer. Information about these and other helpful software is available at:

http://teach.fcps.net/tips/2002_03/October/Cell1

To maintain an affordable production of picture schedules, one may use magazine pictures or photo's taken from the internet to create the schedule. Although software may be easier and beneficial, there may be ways around a lacking budget.

Highlighted Text

It is possible to assist students who struggle with study skills and organization by providing simple, low-tech solutions to their problems. Students who have trouble learning and studying may benefit from using highlighters, markers, colored overlay rulers, or highlighting tape in order to highlight text. This technique is especially useful when reading or studying long texts or passages. These tools can allow for important information to be clearly identified. Some of the highlighting tape available can be written on like a post-it, and can easily be removed if the wrong information has been highlighted. The colored overlay rulers are also readily available, and come in many different colors so students may pick the color that is most appealing to individual needs. The rulers help to reduce glare and provide guidance while reading to aide with tracking. Crossbow education is one company that manufactures and supplies these reading rulers. Students who require extra assistance with organization may benefit from using color coded folders or tabs in order to help with this obstacle. This solution is inexpensive and easy to employ, while making life much easier for the student.

New word processing programs are beginning to integrate a variety of support features in addition to spell-check and thesaurus. One program called WYNN (What You Need Now) is a software tool, created by educators, that incorporates many study strategies to benefit learners with various reading difficulties. Study aids that have been traditionally used with print material have been incorporated, including highlighting, book marking, masking, ruler guides, text or voice annotations and much more. This is a product worth looking into! Making technology part of the writing/publishing process is a must for today's and tomorrow's world.

Recorded Material

Providing students with recorded material to study and learn allows them to listen to and comprehend the content of the text without the stress that may come from reading the information themselves. Auditory learners, as well as those who are visually impaired, may benefit most from this assistive technique. There are many recorders and cassettes available for purchase, which are specifically designed for educational purposes. Many books are available on tape and lectures may also be recorded. There are some companies that, for a reasonable price, will read and record textbooks for use by the student. It is not only beneficial for students to learn by listening to recordings, but to also be able to respond in recorded form. Allowing students to record an essay, as opposed to writing it, may help a student with creativity.

Single Word Scanners

Single word scanners provide complete access to computers or word processing for people who can only use one or more switches. It offers full mouse and keyboard emulation by means of a scanning mode. With each click on the switch the user selects an action, such as move the cursor up or type B, from a "scanning" menu. Scanners are typically used by people who are, for example, quadriplegic due to an accident, or suffering from neuromotor diseases such as Amyotrophic Lateral Sclerosis or Spinal Muscular Atrophy with very limited limb movement.

Pagers

A pager equipped with a vibrator and an alphanumeric display can be used to receive messages. An alphanumeric display is one in which shows letters as well as numbers. The vibrator will signal an incoming message. There is also a paging service available that will allow text messages to be sent from teletype to a pager. These pagers are used primarily to communicate with the deaf or those who are unable to speak

Electronic Organizers

Personal data managers are software packages for computer or electronic handheld device to help with memory and organization. They provide a way to store and retrieve large amounts of personal information easily. You can keep phone numbers, addresses, important dates, appointments, assignments, and reminders in a personal data manager. You enter information using a keyboard or stylus and retrieve it the same way. The information is then displayed on a computer monitor or small liquid crystal display (LCD). Features and capabilities vary a great deal. Some hand-held units connect to a computer to exchange information. Selected hand-held units allow you to enter and retrieve information by speaking into the device, and stored information is spoken back in your own voice.

Voice Output Reminders

Voice output reminders allow for voice recording and playback as well as transcribing features with some voice recognition programs. Date and time stamps and alarms and playback speed are feature to consider. This will help the individual keep track of assignments that are due, or tests that are taking place at a certain time and place.

Software for Concept Development

Software for concept development is a great aid for students with learning, behavior, or cognitive disabilities. Technologies that include strategies of visual organization (e.g. K-W-L) and presentation, image to text connection, and sign language illustration to text connection. Using software to assist in putting concepts together in a visual diagram and then organizing for writing can be a very beneficial strategy for many learners. It can be used to assist learners in becoming literate while having fun. This is a tool for teaching language and literacy skills to students. It quickly pairs pictures with text to help individuals with special needs understand concepts, increase language skills, and develop reading skills. Type in a sentence or story and with one keystroke, it will add the pictures.

Some software programs present an image with each word or group of words. Concepts can be edited to have specific pictures, for example, a picture of a child or staff member. In addition to presenting a story in image/text form, vocabulary cards or cards for Augmentative Communication Devices can be printed. Many products originally created for learners with a variety of learning challenges are becoming successful tools for young and non-literate deaf learners. Graphical information is more commonly found in many products.

Software for Organization of Ideas

Outlining/semantic webbing software can address this precise problem by creating visual-graphic structures to organize ideas, and then convert those visual maps into outlines. These types of programs can be useful for brainstorming ideas and then arranging those ideas into a diagram, which most programs will convert into an outline showing a hierarchy of ideas. Many instructors have used these types of visual maps on newsprint or chalkboards, to demonstrate connections between ideas or to brainstorm ideas. The computer software programs that allow this kind of idea generation are useful for students who need to see and manipulate their ideas. By mapping out ideas, students can easily rearrange them. Then the software program can transform the semantic map into a Roman numeral outline, which may serve to assist the student in developing a draft of an essay. Programs allow users to move, delete, or add ideas at any point in the graphic or numerical outline layout.

Another advantage to using a semantic mapping program is that it can help students avoid getting bogged down in the details of an essay. By mapping out ideas in a graphic way, students are able to stay focused on the main idea and not get lost in irrelevant details. Conversely, for students who have difficulty generating sufficient details to support their main ideas, using a semantic mapping program or integrated writing process software, such as DraftBuilder, could help students see the lack of supportive material.

Hand Held Computers

There are a variety of different hand held computers that can be used for students with disabilities. Personal Digital Assistants (PDA's) is a new technology that is low in cost. They are portable computers that are used for word processing, internet access, calculating, and reading internet websites or files aloud with text-to-speech features. Another other commonly used hand held computer is the calculator.

Part V: Sensory

Section Twelve

VISION

Eyeglasses

Eyeglasses are the most commonly used assistive technology device for students with vision problems. They are easy to handle and are made to precisely assist the students. They help students with both nearsighted and farsighted vision problems. They can be carried with the students at all times throughout the day.

However, students may often be embarrassed to wear their glasses. Teachers need to reinforce to the entire class that glasses are nothing to be ashamed of and they help millions of people with everyday tasks and activities. Teachers may have to remind students to put on their glasses at times, such as when students are going to be watching a movie or completing an assignment. Although it is the primary responsibility of the student to wear his/her glasses, it may be necessary for the teacher to remind the student until he/she becomes adjusted. Glasses are also the most commonly used corrective option for vision problems among American people. Contact lenses are also an option of corrective eye wear for those who prefer to not wear glasses.

Magnifier

When enlarged print is not available to students with vision problems, a magnifier should be provided in order to allow students to readily see print materials. With a magnifier readily available, students with vision problems are able to concentrate on the subject material that is being taught instead of focusing on seeing the words.

Teachers should provide a magnifier to students with vision problems to use throughout the day. The magnifier should be one that the student can easily handle (e.g.—take into consideration fine and gross motor skills) and one that they can keep with them at all times, such as a sheet magnifier.

Large Print Books

The print found in textbooks and books is often small print, which can be difficult to read even by students without vision problems. Since books and textbooks play a large role in daily education, all print information needs to be modified for students with vision problems as much as possible. Without the ability to correctly see the print material, students with vision problems will constantly fall behind and not be able to work to their full potential due to problems outside of their control.

Prior to the beginning of the school year, teachers should make certain that they have textbooks and all tentative books available in large print if they will have a student(s) with vision problems. Placing a student with vision problems next to a student with good vision, patience, and a willingness to help others can also help a student with special needs to succeed in the classroom. Teachers can also use a combination of a magnifier, large print books and non-glare lighting for optimal accommodations for students with vision problems.

Closed Circuit Television (CCT)

A closed circuit television is a video magnification system consisting of a video screen interfaced with a video. This allows students with vision problems to participate in watching television programs that the entire class is watching. A student with vision problems will not have to strain his/her eyes to see the screen and/or sit extremely close to the television screen. The screen allows students to watch something as simple as television with decreased difficulty and without feeling different because of the disability.

When any type of television/video technology is being used in the classroom, accommodations for students with vision problems must be made. Technology is a popular aspect of education that is being strongly integrated into all curricular areas and students with vision problems should be allowed to take advantage of this to the fullest extent. In order for this to happen, teachers need to determine and implement the appropriate and necessary modifications for the student.

Screen Magnifier (Mounted Over the Screen)

In addition to television and video, computers are the most widely used aspect of technology used in education today. They are a necessary way of life and an efficient method for students to use in the learning process. But as with textbooks, the print found on computer screens can be very small. This makes a simple task, such as typing a paper on the computer, extremely difficult.

A screen magnifier is an excellent piece of assistive technology that can be used by students with vision problems. The device goes over the computer screen and the words appear larger so the student can easily read what is on the screen. Once again, this device allows the student to focus on the assignment and not on trying to figure out what is on the screen.

By eliminating some of the obstacles in the learning process, students with disabilities can focus on one task instead of two. This will ultimately lead to increased student performance and interest in learning. Teachers should make certain that students with vision problems should always have their own computer (or laptop) and screen magnifier. Preferential seating, such as placing students with vision problems next to helpful students or closer to the area where information is presented, is a natural accommodation. Additional devices like assistive keyboards, keyboards with larger letter labels, and a mouse can also be beneficial.

Screen Color Contrast

Along with small print, computer screen color poses as another problem for students with vision problems. The bright coloring can be difficult for student to read the words, focus, and can also place strain on the eyes. All of these factors are distractions that can be easily eliminated by contrasting the screen. Students with vision problems can then focus better on the computer screen and the words without having a glare from the coloring. The screen color contrast accommodation should be made in conjunction with the screen magnifier for the best results. It is again the responsibility of the teacher to make certain that this, and all accommodations, are implemented each school day in order for students with vision problems to succeed to the best of their ability.

Screen Reader, Text Recorder

Screen reader is technology that helps to magnify the screen so the user can read what's on the screed more clearly. It also enhances the text using bolding and large print. This type of product is beneficial to individuals who have a wide range of visual impaired requirements. The technology also features text recording, where the individual can hear the on-screen text while using the magnification aspects to enhance learning and reading, thus combining hearing and visual senses.

Braille Materials

Braille is a system of print for the blind which uses raised dots in specific placement to represent letters and words. The raised print is read by feeling with fingers. Individuals with vision problems rely on Braille to maintain a life with all the advantages that people without vision problems live. Technology that allows the person to write in Braille is particularly good for the classroom. Many programs can print to paper or plastic and then emboss the paper. These programs give the student and teacher the chance to communicate with each other on paper.

Braille Translation Software

This type of software is used to translate text into Braille for the visual impaired individual. While it is used to transform text into Braille, it can also be used to convert music into Braille. This is especially important because it allows the person with visual problems to experience all the different types of learning that take place in school, not just the core subjects. This type of software also converts Braille to text, which can be useful to teachers trying to help the visual impaired student to learn.

Enlarged or Braille/Tactile Labels for Keyboard

Braille labels for keyboards enhance typing ability for students with visual problems because the labels are put over the standard keys and the student can then type in Braille with the text remaining the same.

Alternate Keyboard with Enlarged Keys

Keyboards with enlarged keys are for students who have trouble seeing and locating the keys. Enlarged keyboards are larger versions of the standard keyboard and provide an easier target for the student. The keyboards can be in either alphabetic or the standard format, depending on the need of the user. Also, students with visual problems could use enlarged labels for keyboards so it is easier for the students to see the letter without changing the actual keyboard.

Braille Keyboard and Note Taker

This is a keyboard with Braille replacing the standard format for keyboards. It allows the user to type using Braille while producing text. Also, there are devices such as portable note takers that users can bring with them to classrooms or meetings that convert to text and can connect to a computer and print.

Section Thirteen

HEARING

Pen and Paper

Individuals who are deaf or hard of hearing may utilize a pen and paper to assist them when trying to communicate. Those who have trouble speaking can write down their need or want, as well as having the other party write to them to enable communication and understanding. A pen and paper are an example of a low tech assistive device.

Computer/Portable Word Processor

A computer or portable word processor can be especially helpful to individuals who are deaf or hard of hearing. Communication can then take place through typing. The computer has the same purpose as the pen and paper but is higher technology.

TTY/TTD With or Without Delay

The Teletypewriter for the deaf (TTY) or Telecommunications Device for the Deaf (TDD) 'rings' via a flashing light or the more recent vibrating wrist band that resembles a watch. The TTY consists of a keyboard, which holds between 20 and 30 character keys, a display screen, and a modem. The letters that the TTY user types into the machine are turned into electrical signals that can travel over regular telephone lines. When the signals reach their destination (in this case another TTY) they are converted back into letters which appear on a display screen and can be printed out on paper; some TTYs are equipped with answering machines.

Other communication devices that may be used are voice carry over products. These allow the used to speak their end of the conversation, but will allow him/her to receive any response in text format on a display screen. This device needs to be used in conjunction with a Relay Service. Technology also makes it possible for individuals to use video phones, where the user can see the individual who is on the other line; both parties would need to have this type of phone.

Notification Devices

A notification device is used to alert an individual who is deaf or hard of hearing. Some examples may include: visual or vibratory alarm clocks and smoke alarms, telephone and doorbell lights, motion detectors, smoke alarms that give off strong scents to alert. There are a number of other devices available such as wrist watches with alarms, devices that let you know when the baby awakes from their nap, prenatal listening devices, amplified stethoscopes, and many others. New devices are being developed all the time.

Closed Captioning

Individuals who are deaf or hard of hearing benefit from closed captioning programming to understand and enjoy television or videos. Closed-captioning is when words flow across, or pop up on, the screen which matches words or noises in the program. Hardware and software can be purchased to encode captioning in-home. Programs with closed-captioning can be requested from a service bureau. The latter of the two is more time consuming and expensive.

Real Time Captioning

Real time captioning is like captioning for real life. As a person speaks, the words are transcribed and displayed to the audience on a monitor, screen, or laptop computer. This is often used in court houses, news rooms, conferences and in the schools (usually colleges and universities, but its use is even beginning to be seen in elementary schools). When used in an academic setting, the file of the lecture can be made available to the student after their class. The only drawback to this system is that if the speaker goes too fast, the transcription may get behind and skip parts of what was said to catch up.

Computer Aided Note Taking

Computer aided note taking means using a computer to type on a normal computer keyboard to display what is said in a classroom. This system is helpful for students who are not able to hear the lesson. A computer aided note taking device will generate a written transcript in which the student will be able to read.

Flash Alert Signal On Computer

The flash alert signal on a computer is able to alert the user of a change within the computer by flashing the screen instead of alerting with a sound. For a student who has difficulty hearing, this system might alert them to incoming emails, incorrect spelling in documents, weather warnings, and/or upcoming appointments in an agenda.

Phone Amplifier

The phone amplifier is designed for people with mild to moderate hearing loss. It is compact, light weight, and fits easily into a pocket or purse. It has an adjustable volume control of up to 10 times the standard level as well as an automatic tone enhancement for sound clarity. It easily straps onto any standard, cordless, cellular or pay telephone and is hearing aid compatible.

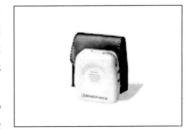

Personal Amplification System/Hearing Aid

A hearing aid is an electronic, battery-operated device that amplifies and changes sound to allow for improved communication. Hearing aids receive sound through a microphone, which then converts the sound waves to electrical signals. The amplifier increases the loudness of the signals and then sends the sound to the ear through a speaker.

FM or Loop System

An FM System is an assistive listening device that improves listening in noise. Signals are transmitted from a talker to the listener by FM radio waves. It uses a remote microphone placed within 6 inches of the desired sound source (usually parent, teacher, or peer). The signal is sent from the microphone to a receiver via radio waves. In individual FM units, a child wears an FM receiver. In sound-field units, all children in a classroom benefit from a receiver/amplifier connected to three or four high fidelity, high frequency emphasis loudspeakers that are positioned around the room.

Infrared System

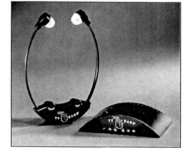

An infrared system is for people with mild to very severe hearing loss who can hear speech but cannot understand the words. Infrared systems are available as wireless headphones that actually raise quiet words above the background sounds and/or music so that the words stand out. There are tone and balance controls which allow you to change the output according to your needs. The user is able to shift the amplification from one ear to the other and from lower to higher frequencies to compensate for different types of hearing loss.

Part VI: Motor

Section Fourteen

CONTROL THE ENVIRONMENT

Introduction

Children and adults with severe disabilities can find it difficult to control their environment. They are often unable to use learning and interactive devices and small appliances. Adding switches and interface devices provide a way for those with disabilities to control their surroundings and learning. The following suggestions and devices help with controlling the environment.

Light Switch Extension

A person in a wheelchair, or someone who cannot extend their arm, may find it difficult to reach a light switch. They may need to have an extension placed on their switch to make it easier to operate. One suggestion is to drill a small hole in the light switch (preferable after the power is cut to the switch), and run a wire through the hole. The next step is to find a small dowel (if the dowel is too large the switch may not remain on) and either put a hole or small eyelet screw in the end. Attach the wire from the switch to the dowel and paint the dowel to match the wall. Commercially made extensions can also be bought, such as the *Light Switch*

Extension Handle. This low tech device includes a flat plastic piece that is attached to the switch plate. It has slots that allow the plastic to move up and down to turn the switch on and off, while the screws of the switch plate hold it in place.

Interface and Switch to Activate Battery Operated Devices

The *Battery Adapter*, by Ablenet, Inc., allows the user to add a switch to a battery operated device. The copper wafer on the product is placed against the positive end of the battery and the toy or device is turned on. The *Switch Latch*, also by Ablenet, Inc., is an interface between the switch and the target device. The toy or device remains on until the switch is pressed again, disconnecting the power to the device. The *Single Switch Latch and Timer*, by Ablenet, Inc., adds a timer to the switch that automatically turns off the device in use.

Interface and Switch to Turn on Electrical Appliances

There are five major kinds of switch interfaces which activate many different types of electrical appliances. The first is an ECU, Environmental Control Unit that serves as an interface for any electrical (DC) appliance with an on / off switch. The second is a Switch–Latch that is connected between the switch and the target device; one touch of the device turns the switch on; the next turns it off. The next one is a timer which connects between the switch and the target device. This device has the ability to run for a set length of time (1-60 seconds) as soon as the switch is activated. More advanced still is the Switch–Latch Timer which offers both features: a timer and latch. This device can be set to turn on a tape player for five seconds. Then the user must re-activate the switch. The fourth type of gadget, a Series Adapter is an interface used between a target device and two switches. Both switches must be activated in order for the device to turn on. The final apparatus, a Jack Adapter converts the size of the switch jack to match the size on the toy or interface.

Radio/Ultra Sound to Remotely Control Appliances

Remote control devices use different methods to operate devices. Two of these methods are ultrasound and radio frequency. Ultrasound uses a high frequency sound wave as the input and output signal. The sound wave will bounce around the room until it reaches the control box and then sends a command signal to the appliance. The input device does not need to be directly aimed at the control box for it to work, but it must be in the same room.

Radio control or radio frequency (RF) is the same that is used in home/car radios as well as garage door openers. An RF system can be used in different rooms but has a limited range of 50-200 feet. So, an input device can be activated from one room (such as the living room) and control an appliance in another room (such as the kitchen or bedroom). Additional wiring is needed in the house or office and interference from another control unit is possible. For example, a neighbor with a garage door opener may be able to turn on/off your lights by simply opening/closing his doors. (http://wata.org/resource/e-control/)

Electronic Aide to Daily Living Controlled Through Augmentative Device

According to the Adaptive Technology Resource Centre (ADTRC), "Electronic Aids for Daily Living (EADL), formerly "Environmental Control Units (ECU)", are simply devices or systems that allow an individual to control facets of their environment. EADL's systems are available as standalone units, or as integrated software using a personal computer. EADL/ECU systems can be controlled by the user in a variety of ways. Some EADL/ECU systems are voice activated, and others are switch activated." Such devices include:

- *Voice Activated Environmental Control Unit,* by Quartet Technology, Inc., which recognizes voice commands for activating devices.
- The *Switch Activated Environmental Control Unit*, also by Quartet Technology, Inc., allows users to control their environment with any one of dozens of skill switches, such as pneumatic or button/key pads.
- *Ultra One,* by Tash, Inc., provides a one touch switch to activate appliances.
- *ActiveHome*, by X10 Wireless Technology, Inc., allows the user to set timers for lighting and appliances from their computer.
- Infra-Link *"Elevator Control"* allows the disabled person to activate elevators doors and the inside controls.
- *Cintex3* is a voice operated device that can be used with voice recognition systems to control the environment. Telephones, TV's, CD players, lamps, and fans can be controlled without the use of hands.

Section Fifteen

POSITIONING AND SEATING

Non-slip Surface on Chair

Assistive technology for positioning and seating can be as simple as having the correct size chair and correct height table. It can also include more complex, custom made items that address a child's very unique needs. The most important thing to remember is that no one can function effectively if they are not well positioned. Dycem is a company that specializes in medical equipment and their non-slip, foam products such as the rubber mat. They are commonly used for chairs used by students with special needs.

Custom Fitted Wheelchair or Insert

Making sure that a student is provided with a comfortable wheelchair is critical for achieving maximum stability and performance. When a student is provided with this comfort and security, he or she will function better at all tasks. There are a wide variety of wheelchairs and insert cushions available to provide for the varying needs of each individual student. Some of these are specifically designed to prevent sores and discomfort that may result from prolonged restriction to a wheelchair. Posture may also be helped by these inserts.

Bolster Seats

Bolster seats are used to provide mobility-impaired persons with greater body stability, maintain upright posture, provide trunk/head support, and reduction of pressure to the skin. Be sure to use proper seat belt for safety.

Rolled Towel

Rolled towels are used to keep young backs straight and allow a child to reach the mouse and keyboard without stretching unnaturally. Rolled towels can be secured by using masking tape. It is very cost effective and yet easy to provide instant support.

Blocks for Feet

Blocks for feet are used to provide stability for someone who has trouble standing up out of a wheelchair or any other sitting position. The blocks will add support to the lower levels of the body and give the individual a boost while rising. An example of low cost blocks for feet is a 3 ring binder.

Adapted/alternate Chair, Side Layer, Stander

Any time a student has difficulties with mobility or stability when seated, adapted/alternate chairs, side layers, and standers need to be considered. They are critical for access to the educational program. An adapted/alternate chair provides multiple adjustments and options to accommodate special needs. The seat adjusts in depth/height and each armrest is height adjustable and swings out for easy entry. The chair even comes complete with armrests and a seat belt.

Side layers are used to position children easily when they are lying down. A student with special needs can lie on their left or right side in a secure comfortable position. The side layers even come with two padded seatbelts that adjust for the girth of a child as well as the height of a child.

Lastly, a stander is used to help a child stand and it allows the child to move independently. It provides children with support and weight bearing through the lower extremities with posterior support. Overall, these types of assistive technologies may allow the student greater access to the educational activities.

http://www.specialkidszone.com/Product_Level1.asp?CategoryID=31

Section Sixteen

MOBILITY

Walker

A walker is an excellent form of assistance for any student with mobility problems such as limping, growth problems, broken bones, etc. This device allows students to move around using their muscles and not be confined to a wheelchair. These students have limited mobility, but are able to manage walking with assistance. A walker can be easily used to move on most surfaces, and can be a long or short term type of assistance. Teachers need to make certain that students with a walker have adequate space in the classroom and hallway to move freely and have the necessary accommodations throughout the classroom. Walkers can be specially made and should be customized to meet the individual needs of the student.

Grab Bars and Rails

Grab bars and rails should be used for students who have a less severe form of mobility problems. These students may simply take a longer time to walk in the hallway due to growth problems, weakened ability to move joints and muscles, and/

or recently had a broken or sprained leg or ankle. They need assistance in moving long distances and do not have much control of their balance. Grab bars and rails allow students to move with assistance but without having to use a walker. These devices should be set up in the classroom and in the hallway to allow students to move with assistance throughout the classroom and the school building. Some grab bars and rails are permanently placed to accommodate all students, while some can be removed to assist students as they are moving along from one destination to the next.

Manual Wheelchair Including Sports Chair

Those students with severe mobility problems are confined to a wheelchair and need much assistance throughout their school day. Manual wheelchairs are difficult to move and require much strength and coordination on the part of the user. Therefore, this type of chair is best used by students with good upper mobility. Manual wheelchairs have changed much over the last couple decades and come in many styles and types to fit a variety of needs and accommodations. Sports chairs are lightweight and are a preferred method by most people requiring additional assistance. A variation of the sports chair is the three-wheeled chair which is used to play sports, such as tennis and basketball with assistance. While the majority of manual wheelchairs tend to be large and bulky, teachers need to make the necessary accommodations throughout the classroom on a daily basis, including desk arrangements, hallways arrangements, doorway and walkway traffic and the ability to move around the school building. Many schools are not equipped to accommodate students in wheelchairs, so it is necessary to make certain that students in this type of situation receive the accommodations they deserve as part of their education.

Powered Mobility Toy

The powered mobility toy is a battery-powered base that is used with an adjustable positioning frame that can support the individual who is standing. The individual can then drive the powered mobility toy by standing, using a joystick. It is designed to give greater mobility to children who have difficulty using a powered wheelchair. The seat can be adjusted depending on the need of the individual, whether it's reclining or standing more upright. The control joystick also can vary depending on the need of the user, and it can also be repositioned to give the user more comfortable access.

Powered Scooter

Powered scooters are battery powered, three or four wheel machines, which allow for greater mobility by users. There are many different styles of powered scooters. It depends on the preference of the user as to what features the scooter will have. The machines vary on size, speed, and storage space. These machines can be very useful for individuals with mobility difficulty. It allows the user to have access to areas the person may not have had access to previously. Powered scooters are controlled by a steering device and individuals who use the scooters generally are not as physically impaired as individual who need a powered wheelchair. The individual generally sits on stool/seat connected to the scooter and that person must step up on the machine in order to use the scooter.

Powered Wheelchair

Powered wheelchairs are battery-powered machines that allow for greater mobility to the user. The powered wheelchairs are very useful for individuals who have difficulty moving their arms as well mobility difficulty. It is for individuals who are more physically impaired than users of powered scooters. The powered wheelchairs vary in size, power, and features depending on the need of the individual. Some factors that must be considered when selecting a powered wheelchair are the individual's physical feature, functioning ability, and usage requirements. Also, the style of wheelchair must fit the lifestyle of the individual. The user must ask the question on where it will be used, whether that's at home, school, or work.

Adapted Vehicle for Driving

This type of Assistive technology gives individuals the opportunity to drive. The types of devices vary depending on the needs of the individual. Some examples of adaptations to vehicles are varying hand controls, left foot gas pedal, pedal extensions for brake, gas and clutch, and driver seat adaptation. Hand controls can give a person access to the pedals without having to use their feet. Driver seat adaptation brings the individual closer to the steering wheel or a gives the user the ability to see out of the front and rear windows. Also, individuals who cannot drive but still need access to vehicles can use wheelchair lifts and ramps that can be customized to fit the vehicle. Many types of vans can be customized to give individuals access to vehicles. As with the powered wheelchair, the individual must evaluate their needs and determine which device would best fit their lifestyle.

Manual Wheelchairs. http://www.abledata.com/text2/manwhch.htm

Section Seventeen

ACTIVITIES OF DAILY LIVING (ADLS)

Introduction

Devices for Activities of Daily Living (ADL) enable the arthritic and others with reduced dexterity, disabled, and elderly to perform activities of daily living, which ordinarily they would have difficulty doing by themselves.

Non-slip Materials
In the area of non-slip materials, there are three manufacturers who lead the innovation: Atstar, Dysem, and Care4u. This form of assistive technology could provide greater independence for the aforementioned groups. As defined, non-slip materials work to hold items firm and securely in place.

Anti-slip mats can be positioned under household objects in order to prevent slipping or spilling for people with disabilities. For example, these mats could be positioned under dishes, bowls, phones, calculators, writing paper, pet bowls, and even remote controls. The companies also sell jar openers made of non-slip material. The material also provides a secure base for floor exercises, and can help carpets to remain in place. An important benefit of this product is that the mats do not adhere to the surface onto which they are placed, therefore making them portable.

Universal Cuff/Strap that Holds Items In Hand

Items that help with control of the environment are devices that a person can turn on or off. They are electronic devices with a special switch or tool. They are sometimes called "Electronic Aids for Daily Living" or EADLs. They are, in general, more "high tech" than the items mentioned above.

Aids for ADL are the many devices that help us with daily routine activities such as eating, cooking, and dressing. Most of these are "low tech" devices that are very inexpensive but they can make a big difference in an individual's independence. The universal cuff strap offers independence for lifting and controlling small motor movements. They also give the ability to hold on to any common device used for daily living. A child could utilize the universal cuff to pick up, hold, and color with a crayon. An adult could use an extended arm to help them get dressed, prepare a simple meal, or brush their teeth.

Color Coded Items for Easier Locating

Color coding can be helpful to people with organizational and cognitive impairments. The following list gives helpful suggestions for the use of color coding in daily living.

- Equipment with numerous controls and multiple functions may be confusing for some people. Shields and color codes placed on those controls that are not required for individual use are helpful.
- Help define the tub by placing light colored mats in dark tubs, and dark colored mats in light tubs to identify the bottom of the tub and bring it closer.
- Paint door trims along hallways in contrasting colors to make identification easier; bathroom trim blue, bedroom trim yellow, etc.
- Color code frequently used items, i.e., edibles like sugar, pudding, and cream are color coded blue; cleaning supplies are color coded red; personal care products like toothpaste, shampoo, and eye drops are color coded yellow.

- Attach brightly colored labels to materials that are hot, poisonous, flammable, or otherwise dangerous to identify products that are "off limits."
- Color code kitchen measuring cups and spoons for easy recipe reading.
- Colored files or file tabs help keep important or frequently used papers organized and readily available.

Adaptive Eating Utensils

These items can be used to assist children in grasping utensils so they can concentrate on learning self-feeding skills. They can be purchased or homemade. Below is one example.

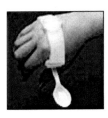

Eating can be an exhausting endeavor for any person with physical disabilities, such as Cerebral Palsy or various degrees of paralysis. The invention of Velcro and its relationship with Adaptive Technology has increased the practicability and economic advantage to purchased or homemade devices. There are utensils designed for an easy and comfortable grip, such as, straight cutlery with built up handles that are combined with a 9" inner lip plate.

Adaptive Drinking Devices

As well as eating, drinking is a huge challenge for people with disabilities. Drinking container options are determined through assessment of the individual and his/her needs.

Grips, handles, length, width size, and material are some considerations used to set the person with the disability with the correct device. Two options available through catalog are:

- Adaptive drinking devices (e.g. cup with cut out rim)
- 10oz. clear double handled mug with mouth piece lid.

**See below pictures for illustrations of adaptive drinking devices.

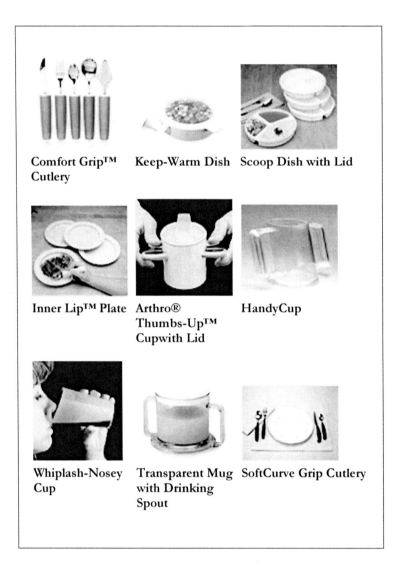

Adaptive Dressing Equipment

Stiffness, pain, weakness, or paralysis can make dressing and undressing particularly difficult. Adaptive dressing equipment can help relieve some of the pain, discomfort, and problems associated with physical disabilities.

Activities of Daily Living (ADLs)   87

Velcro can be very useful when it comes to dressing. The Velcro fastener can help people who have problems with items such as buttons and zippers. Also, Velcro can aid in fastening shoes that can not be tied or reached.

Florida Alliance for Assistive Services and Technology (http://faast.org/atresources/clothing.htm) has a booklet which gives many helpful suggestions for people needing help with dressing. Some of the suggestions are:

- Sew cuff buttons on with elastic thread; keep them buttoned all the time and simply slide your hand through.
- Remove buttons from the cuff or front of a blouse or shirt, and sew the button to the closed buttonhole borders. Sew Velcro on the two sides and press to close.
- Attach a ring or loop to the zipper tab so it's easier to catch with fingers or a dressing aid.
- Sew loops or tabs of ribbon or seam blinking inside clothes to help in pulling them on or off.
- Adapt a brassiere by sewing up the back closure, cutting the front open, and attaching Velcro strips.
- To keep a shirt or blouse tucked in, sew rubber strips to the inside of your skirt or slacks waistband.
- Slacks can be fitted with side zippering in the legs to ease in pulling them on and off. Zippers in the inside seam to the knee may accommodate a cast or brace.
- Other devises for purchase include button hooks and sock assistants to help with independent dressing. Medical supply companies are a good source for such devices.

Adaptive Devices for Hygiene

Several devices are available for hygienic care. These devices are helpful for seniors and the disabled to maintain their independence. Many of these products help with range of motion, coordination, and gross motor difficulties.

Pistol Grip Remote Toe Nail Clipper has a long handle that make clipping toenails possible with very little bending. This product can be useful to people who are pregnant, overweight, or those with back pain. The *Table Top Nail Clippers,* by Dynamic Living, also allows the user to clip finger nails with a secure, non-slip, device.

Long Handle Brushes and Combs allow people with limited range of motion to care for their own hair.

Soapy Soles clean and massage feet without having to reach down and balance in the shower or tub. Feet do not need to be raised in order to become clean.

Nail Brush with suction cup base allows the finger nails to be cleaned with one hand. The suction cups allow the brush to remain stable. The brush can also be used as a vegetable cleaner in the kitchen.

NAIS makes a personal hygiene system, or bidet. This device can be attached to the toilet in place of the regular seat. The bidet allows the user to clean his or herself without the use of toilet tissue. Other adaptive toilet seats provide elevation to the seat to make it easier to sit and stand.

Snap and Roll allows a person to change the toilet paper with one hand and in one easy motion.

Adaptive Bathing Devices

Products for assistance with bathing come in many forms. There are devices that help with entry and exit from bathing areas, the bathing itself, and safety while bathing. The products can help a person feel independent in caring for their personal needs. The following are only a few of the available adaptive devices that can be used in bathing.

Shower head extenders can assist people with disabilities by allowing them to control the aim and flow of the water. These devices are available at most hardware and large department stores.

Maddawash terry soap mitts provide a "palm pocket" to hold a bar of soap. This can be used for bathing or for washing dishes.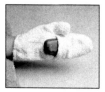

Transfer benches, such as the one seen here from Care4u Senior Resources, allow the bather to enter the bathtub by sitting on the bench and sliding across the tub rim.

Grab bars in the tub, shower, and near the toilet help the individual to safely move around the bathroom. Many hardware stores and medical supply companies have a variety of these devices to choose from.

No Rinse shampoo allows the bather to wash their hair without water. There is also a No Rinse shampoo cap available. These products are ideal for those who cannot get into a shower or bath.

Back scrubbers come in many styles and shapes. They can assist the bather in reaching the back.

Sponge on a Stick, available from Dynamic Living, provides a more comfortable method of washing the back and lower extremities for people with reduced range of motion.

Adaptive Equipment for Cooking

There are many products on the market to aid in cooking. Many aids can be adapted from everyday items instead of specially purchased equipment. The following is a partial list of equipment that can be used in the kitchen to help people with disabilities.

- Mirror over stove so you can see into pots from your wheelchair.
- Special tools to open jars.
- Special reaching tools (called "reachers") to help you pick up things that are too far away.
- Tenodesis splint to help you pick up tiny objects when you don't have a strong pinch.
- Prism glasses so you can look straight down if you can't bend your neck forward.
- Mouthsticks are useful to those who cannot move their hands at all.
- Toaster ovens to provide accessibility and flexible cooking areas
- Bowl Holders: this device grips a bowl firmly while you stir batter and other foods

- Nail Board: this is a simple wooden cutting board with two upright nails on it used to secure food so it can be cut with one hand.
- Rocking Knives: an inexpensive tool that makes it easy to prepare and cut food at mealtime.

Section Eighteen

RECREATION

Toys Adapted With Velcro, Magnets, Handles, Etc.

Play is an integral part of children's development, enabling them to purposefully interact with their environment. Toys are tools for socialization. Due to limited motor ability, many children with disabilities are passive observers and are unable to independently play with toys. Their attempts to play can turn a potentially pleasurable activity into a frustrating experience. Thanks to modern technology, many toys can be adapted so that children with disabilities can use them. Small handles and knobs on toys such as Magna Doodle can be extended with PVC tubes, hollow dowels or rubber tubing (the kind used for making fishing rod handles). Velcro is of course invaluable. Other types of toys that can be easily accessed are those that are sound or motion activated. This type of toy encourages sound production and purposeful movement. By using handle extenders, many of the popular toys found in local toy stores or some that will be available through KidNeeds.com can be adapted and enjoyed by children and their siblings or peers.

Toys Adapted For Single Switch Operation

Most battery toys can be adapted for use with interchangeable switches that can be activated with any part of the body that has purposeful movement. These toys are useful for children who cannot use toys normally but can operate a simple switch. This can be done, in most cases, with a simple to make battery interrupter. Single switch cd-roms are also available for students.

Adaptive Sporting Equipment

There is adaptive sporting equipment for people who want to paint, draw, dance, sing, act, build, hunt, fish, hike, water ski, rock climb, canoe, camp, play golf, garden or lift weights. There is a tree stand for hunters, automated fishing equipment, water skis for folks in wheelchairs. Some of the equipment is expensive, but others can be made with things you have laying around the house. Providing this adaptive equipment may increase the quality of life for individuals with disabilities.

Universal Cuff

The Universal Cuff may be used with a crayon or paint brush to help an individual with low muscle tone use the utensil independently. This device wraps around the palm and back of hand to enable the user to hold the utensil.

Modified Utensils

Utensils can be modified in many ways to provide assistance to those individuals who need extra help in accomplishing daily functions. These modifications can range in cost from the very inexpensive exercise grips for crayons or markers to the very expensive exercise animatronics computerized arms that are designed to complete the function they are programmed to do.

Arm and Wrist Supports

Arm support devices stabilize and support arms and wrists while the user is typing or using a mouse or trackball. The wrist rests support the wrist while using a keyboard. Potential users are people who need additional support to avoid fatigue or pain and also benefit from having arms stabilized. Some features to consider are provided support at the arm or wrist. Some supports attach to the table in front of the drawing surface. Some have cuffs to support the forearm, adjustable heights, swivel in two or more directions, and mount on the chair instead of the table. One or both arms can also be supported in a variety of ways, depending on individual preference. Before the release of commercial products, people used foam wedges or foam bars to supply the support needed.

Electronic Aids to Operate TV, VCR, ETC.

One electronic aid that is used to assist individuals with limited vision and memory/organization is the Large Button Universal Remote. The large buttons on the remote make it easier for people to locate and identify what they are pushing. The large button universal remote may also be helpful for some individuals with limited hand use. A remote control unit is also helpful for users with limited reaching/lifting and mobility/balance who may be unable to access the TV or VCR itself.

The Sony Dream Machine with Remote is an AM/FM stereo clock radio with a built-in CD player. It comes with a 4 button remote control that is used to control the snooze button, the radio, the CD player, and to turn the machine on/off. The simplified remote control provides an easy way to turn on/off your favorite CD or preset radio station for users with limited memory/organization and vision. The remote control is useful for individuals with limited mobility/balance and reaching/lifting, who may be unable to access the unit itself.

Art Software

There is a variety of assistive art software used for children. A few types of the software are Disney's Magic Artist, Art Dabbler, and Kid Pix Studio Deluxe. Disney's Magic Artist is recommended for children ages 5–12. It includes animated traditional art tools and wacky tools. It also includes natural media simulation, fun sound effects, colorful backgrounds and Disney stamps. Disney's Magic Artist has larger color squares than KidPix so it would be better to use for a student who has visual problems. Kid Pix has a text-to-speech function, sound, and special effects, which is great for kids. Children using Kid Pix have the ability to edit or create their own stamp clip art. Kid Pix is also available in Spanish and English. Art Dabbler is the next step up from Kid Pix because it has more technical capability. It also has more sophisticated tools and still retains sound effects.

Games on the Computer

Games on the computer which can be controlled by a variety of standard and adaptive technology methods are designed for children and adults with disabilities. These methods include expanded keyboards, headmouse and joysticks which make it possible to play a game with a single switch. For example, Alien Invasion, Ruby Ridge and Brickout are games which can be adjusted for players with a very wide range of abilities. These level games are designed to be accessible for players who are unable to handle the high-speed and rapid-fire pace of traditional computer games. You can download these games for free via the internet at www.arcess.com.

Part VII: Top Ten

Section Nineteen

APPROXIMATELY $1 TOOLBOX

Rubber Band

The device for under $1 that will be looked at is a rubber band that can be used as a grip for pens and pencils. This type of assistive technology is for any individual with difficulty holding writing instruments. The user has a problem gripping a pen or pencil and thus has hard time writing. This type of assistive technology is very easy to use. The individual that is using the rubber band wraps the item just below the area where the person grips the writing utensil. The user must wrap the rubber band until it is tight and does not slip off. The user then writes with the pen or pencil in a normal way and has greater control over the instrument without slippage because the user has a rubber surface to hold on to. The individual can use the rubber band pen/pencil grip whenever he or she has to write. It is especially useful in the classroom or meetings when it is necessary to write. It is also very good when the individual has to write for a prolonged time, such writing essays for an exam or taking notes in class.

The rubber band grip is an inexpensive and effective way for an individual with difficulty holding on to a pen or pencil to grip the writing instrument. It gives the user the ability to write without having to worry about constant interruption because of their inability to grip a pen or pencil for extended periods of time. The rubber band can be used wherever the individual needs it. It is portable and can fit into a person's pocket. Also, once the device is put on the pen or pencil, there is no reason to remove it until that pen or pencil needs to be replaced.

A disadvantage of the device is how small the item is and it can easily be lost. Also, if it is attached to a pen or pencil, and you lose the writing utensil, you lose the device if it is still connected. But this problem does not take away from the effectiveness of the product, and it can be replaced for a very small amount of money. One other disadvantage that may arise from the rubber band grip is the durability of the band. Often, rubber bands are prone to snapping and, depending on use, the device could weaken and break. But, as previously stated, the inexpensive nature of this product does make it easy to replace.

Clipboard

A tool used to assist students with poor fine and gross motor skills that is very useful is a clipboard. This device is used by placing paper on top of a strong board to have a better grip while writing. The clipboard is very user-friendly; any student can use this device. It is used so students do not have to hold their paper steadily while writing. It also helps when students are doing work at a seat other than their desk. A clipboard can be transported anywhere and is accommodating for students of all ages.

Pen/Pencil Grip

A tool used to assist students with poor fine and gross motor skills and writing difficulties is a pen/pencil grip. It consists of a soft/rubbery material that goes over the section of the writing instrument where the fingers are in order to provide support and coordination while writing. It can be used each time a student writes. The purpose is to help ease with writing. The device can be taken everywhere with the student and is applicable for students of all ages.

Sponge

A sponge can be used as a means of support for students with joint and muscle problems to make writing easier. One sponge can be placed under the wrist area of the student and serves as a cushion while writing. It can be used each time a student writes. The purpose is to provide comfort and ease while writing. It should be used in conjunction with a clipboard, pen/pencil grip, etc. to provide maximum support. The device can be taken everywhere with the student and is applicable for students of all ages.

3 Ring Binders

A three ring binder can be used as a support to provide a level surface for writing. It is for individuals with writing difficulties and for people with hand to eye coordination problems. The individual uses the device by setting it down on a flat surface and puts the paper they are writing on top of the binder. The 3 ring binder can be used anytime the individual needs to write, whether it's in the classroom or at home. It is important to use because the individual may have difficulty writing on a flat surface. The slant of the 3 ring binder provides the individual with the flat surface that is necessary for the person to be able to write properly. The 3 ring binder is portable and can fit easily into any bag, which can be brought wherever the user needs it. One disadvantage of the 3 ring binder is its durability. The binder can collapse easily and is also prone to ripping with extended use.

Tongs

Tongs can be used by individuals that have difficulty reaching everyday items. The tongs can be simple cooking tongs generally used to flip different types of foods. The tongs can be used by any person who can't reach items or who may have difficulty gripping things. The tongs are very easy to use because the individual grips the tongs with one hand, much like scissors. The tongs can be used whenever an individual has difficulty reaching or gripping an item. The benefit is that the tongs give the user access to items they might not have originally been able to reach. The tongs are not very large and can be placed in any type of bag, making them very portable.

Cloth Grip

A cloth grip can be used by individuals that must use a walker or rails. Often when using these items, the hands become sweaty and can be prone to slippage. The cloth is wrapped around the walker where the individual holds it and the user grips the cloth. Thus, the user is less likely to lose hold of the walker and fall. The cloth grip can be placed on any walker or rail and is easy to assemble. The cloth grip is needed because there is no fiction between the hand and the metal bar where the user holds on to the walker, which causes slippage. One disadvantage of the cloth grip is that the user may need to replace it occasionally after it has been worn out through use. Due to the inexpensive nature of the product, it is easily replaced.

Tennis Balls

Tennis ball(s) are another accessory than can be used with a walker. The tennis ball(s) is placed on the bottom of the walker and allows the user to move more smoothly without having to stop. Normally when using a walker, the individual must stop after every step to lift the walker. Using the tennis ball(s) on the bottom allows the user to glide along the surface and not have to stop after each step to lift the walker. The tennis ball(s) can be used whenever or wherever the individual goes with the walker. This item is important to use because it increases movement for individuals that need a walker by decreasing the amount of lifting necessary when using it. A disadvantage of the item is the tennis ball(s) can wear out easily.

Stress Ball

A stress ball can be used by individuals to help increase muscle movement in their hands and wrists. The individual squeezes on the stress ball repeatedly to increase muscle strength and coordination. This type of exercise is especially effective for individuals with difficulty gripping items or holding on to items. The stress ball can be used practically anywhere at any time. Whenever the individual is not doing much, they could squeeze the stress ball. The item is small enough to fit into a pocket and can travel wherever the user goes.

Section Twenty

RESOURCES

Bowser, G., & Reed, P. (1998). Education Tech Points: A Framework for Assistive Technology Planning. Winchester, OR: CATO: P.O. Box 431, Winchester, OR 97495; www.edtechpoints.org

> This manual uses six points to aid technology planning. Each Education Tech Point identifies the specific times within the planning and provision of specially designed instruction that the need for assistive technology (both devices and services) should be considered. Education Tech Points offer a way to integrate assistive technology into the thinking of the Individualized Education Planning team and the management system that each school district uses to ensure provision of appropriate services to children with disabilities.

Golden, D. (1998). Assistive Technology in Special Education: Policy and Practice. Council of Administrators of Special Education, Fort Valley State University, 1005 State University Drive, Fort Valley, GA 31030

Reed, P. (Ed.). (2000). Assessing Students' Need for Assistive Technology. Oshkosh, WI: WATI; www.wati.org

> The mission of the Wisconsin Assistive Technology Initiative (WATI) isto ensure that every child in Wisconsin who needs assistive technology (AT) will have equal and timely access to an appropriate evaluation and the provision and implementation of any needed AT devices and services. A primary goal is to improve the outcomes and results for children and youth with disabilities through the use of assistive technology to access school programs and curriculum. The project is designed to increase the capacity of school districts to provide assistive technology services by making training and technical assistance available to teachers, therapists, administrators and parents throughout Wisconsin.

Reed, P., & Bowser, G. (2000). Assistive Technology Pointers for Parents. Winchester, OR: CATO; www.edtechpoints.org

> Assistive Technology Pointers for Parents includes a workbook to help parents work with schools and other agencies to identify appropriate assistive technology. In this workbook there are many real life stories which illustrate the use of the Education Tech Points Framework in identifying assistive, acquiring and using assistive technology for a particular child. Stories about real children help to illustrate the important role that parents play on the assistive technology team.

Bowser, G., & Reed, P. (1998). Education Tech Points: A Framework for Assistive Technology Planning. Winchester, OR: CATO; P.O. Box 431, Winchester, OR 97495; www.edtechpoints.org

Golden, D. (1998). Assistive Technology in Special Education: Policy and Practice. Council of Administrators of Special Education, Fort Valley State University, 1005 State University Drive, Fort Valley, GA 31030

Reed, P. (Ed.). (2000). Assessing Students' Need for Assistive Technology. Oshkosh, WI: WATI; www.wati.org

Reed, P., & Bowser, G. (2000). Assistive Technology Pointers for Parents. Winchester, OR: CATO; www.edtechpoints.org

Journal And Newsletter

Closing the Gap, P.O. Box 68, Henderson, MN 65044
www.closingthegap.com

Journal of Special Education Technology, Free with TAM Membership (a division of CEC); jset.unlv.edu

Special Education Technology Practice, Knowledge by Design, 5907 N. Kent Ave., Whitefish Bay, WI 53217-4615; www.setp.net

Internet Sites

http://www.teachertube.com/index.php
http://www.abilityhub.com/links/organization.htm
http://www.nockonline.org/?gclid=CIb1s8Kdp5QCFSgZHgod-xt2tw
http://www2.edc.org/fsc/www.closingthegap.com-- Searchable database of AT plus articles from their newsletter.
www.fctd.info-- Family Center on Technology and Disability. Extensive AT Resource reviews, user-friendly resource library and more.
www.LDonline.com-- Section on AT. To get to it, go to LD In Depth and then Technology.
www.tamcec.org-- The website of the Technology and Media Division of CEC.
Trace.wisc.edu- Links to adaptive freeware and shareware for computer access.
www.wati.org- Wisconsin Assistive Technology Initiative has WATI assessment forms, updates, lending library, information, best practice tips, and more